More

Laughing

D1569219

and

Loving

with

Autism--

A collection of "real life" warm and humorous stories

R. Wayne Gilpin

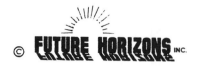

Dedication

There are many who deserve recognition for this book but clearly the parents, families and friends of children and adults with autism are the real authors and heroes in the challenge of autism.

Then, there is Alex, my son. My time with him in his 15 years has taught me volumes about myself, my limits and the joy of unqualified love. His unique perspective of the world and his efforts to be better have earned my respect.

Next, but no less important, to my daughter Jennifer, who is often normal but never boring. Then, there is my business partner, Polly, who has accepted the time given to this book and the Autism Society with grace and patience.

Finally, to my sister Dorothy, who would have loved this book. I like to think that somewhere, in a better place, she is enjoying the stories about her nephew, and smiling.

Introduction

To those of you not familiar with autism, let me explain what it is, and isn't, in very basic terms. It is not life threatening, rarely dangerous to others in any way and can't be "given" to anyone.

Autism is a developmental and communication disorder that acts as a block to "normal" interaction. It's as if a wall drops down around the autistic that interferes with the ability to communicate, feel or understand in "normal" ways. Nuances or subtleties are often lost on a child with autism because it requires too much in-depth understanding.

Where we understand a story or activity because of its "meaning", they listen to the words and their literal interpretation. This "negative" is the basis for a lot of the humor--they see things exactly as they are offered. In doing so, they often illustrate our own too serious view of the same words or act.

It's also worth adding that the word autism covers everything from those who are non-verbal and self-injurious to a few that graduate from college but still have serious problems applying skills because of the "communication wall."

There have been many books written on autism by knowledgeable professionals who have explored causes, "cures" and treatments of autism. Many of them had the first name of "Doctor" and have written with great depth and use of medical terms attempting to define and treat this mysterious disorder. Others have written from the perspective of the autistic or a family member. They have all, and usually with great skill, written in very serious terms about an admittedly serious subject.

However, if you want a book that labors on the pain of autism, you're holding the wrong book. This writing emphasizes the unique views that persons with autism have of us, our values, our words and the things we feel are so serious. In fact, very often the humor is found in how they illuminate our "proprieties" and structured attitudes. A person with autism simply sees the obvious and relates to that image without being "hampered" by rules of our society. They see a world consumed by "saying the right thing." This gives them the freedom to see everything literally, and to speak honesty when we normal people would hold our tongues.

No one questions that all parents of autistic children would prefer to have the handicap removed. Yet no parent, sibling, teacher or friend does not balance that desire by drawing comfort from the love and laughter that gives us strength. We share the following anecdotes and stories so you can feel the positives of this challenge, and the joys that our "handicapped" loves bring to our lives.

This is a book intended to be a source of smiles, laughter, sharing and maybe a few warm tears.

The Reaction

It was a "fun" idea..

"Wayne, why don't you write a book on all the funny stories about Alex?".....Hey, Wayne, what's the latest on Alex?"......"I told the last story about Alex to my college class and they loved it!"

Slowly, the concept of writing a book on Alex's view of life and his humorous perspectives began to formulate. However, as I related my plans to other parents and teachers, they would smile and say, "great idea, reminds me of what Jason did the other day," or, "God, yes, the other day my daughter blew me away when she....."

I then realized that the wonderful asset of humor in autism was not at all unique to my son, but to virtually all children and adults with autism. Therefore, I decided to request others who interacted with children and adults with autism to join me in offering the humorous, lighter side of autism to the world.

At first, the stories came in slowly; some poorly written, yet very funny, others perfectly composed. There were others that, certainly unintentionally, seemingly poked fun at the child. This went against my intent, which was to show their wonderful innocence and literal view of life, the very factors that often demonstrated our own folly.

Some were not at all funny and were not intended to be. Rather, they spoke of progress, strength and courage. At first, I put them on the side as my book was intended to be only humorous. However, I was continually drawn back to that group of letters and finally included them under a chapter headed "poignant", as I realized that elements of progress, no matter how measured, and courage are the very components that allow us the emotional room to enjoy the humor.

It took far more time and effort than I had imagined, but as the book molded, I was sure that here was a source of comfort, enjoyment, smiles, and tears that would leave parents or teachers of a child with autism feeling better after reading it rather than feeling defeated.

I thought, "Good little book; we'll print 500, hope our little publishing company doesn't lose too much money on it and the Autism Society of America can realize a few dollars in royalties." I dramatically underestimated the impact.

"Laughing and Loving.." was introduced at the International Conference on Autism in Canada and, to our shock, outsold virtually every book there!

One mother came up to our booth and hugged me as she related how good it made her feel. She was immediately followed by a woman of over six feet who gave me a very aggressive handshake and said, "Good going, Gilpin, (I had never met the woman) that's the best damn bathroom book I've ever read! Now, all my guests will feel better about autism when they use **the room**". I THINK she was offering a compliment.

The response from parents and teachers was greater than we had expected, but the real surprise was that parents of "normal" children bought and enjoyed "Laughing and Loving with Autism." Then colleges began ordering the book for their psychology and mental health classes. Professors were calling in saying that it explained, in a "user friendly" way, how those with autism viewed the world. As one teacher sagely put it, "I'm using it for my class for three reasons. First, it gives a refreshing view of autism. Secondly, I know they'll read it because it"s funny, and third--it's only $9.95!" All sounded like pretty good reasons to me.

Additionally, the book was reviewed in six different newspapers, including three nearly full page stories on Alex and my daughter Jennifer (who wrote the best piece in the book). Finally, I did three radio talk shows and two television programs answering questions from an interested, but generally misinformed audiences.

I never planned to write, or, more accurately, compile a sequel. However, reader response coupled with a flood of new, funny and touching stories gently coerced me into another labor of love.

Relax and enjoy!

I've wondered if all the Jerry Lewis characters were, in fact, high functioning young men with autism... Think about it! By now, autisic behavior could be very popular in France.

Laughing

Many of the stories are about my son Alex and I've put those in this typeface. In this way, you can trace common trends in his vision of our world. All other stories are followed by the name of the person who so graciously offered the anecdote. For the most part, the stories are in their own words.

As mentioned earlier, no one questions the challenge of autism. However, it is equally true that these children and adults can suddenly offer a ray of humor that brightens our day. These offerings are representative of the humor "from left field" that often brings us back to the reality of their perspective.

Laughing

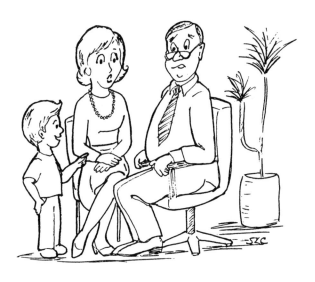

"Be Careful What You Ask..."

It was to be a very big day. I was taking my son, James, to one of the leading experts on auditory training in Canada, Dr. Binet. Because I was to have an appointment with this highly regarded doctor, several of the aides who work with James asked if they could accompany me so they could meet this well-known expert in the field of autism. We all excitedly prepared for this big day and drove the several hour trip to his office. Our group of four, the two aides, James and myself went in to meet the doctor somewhat apprehensively. Dr. Binet was very gracious as he sensed our nervousness, speaking first to me and then to the aides as he asked and answered questions.

Suddenly, he turned to James and said, "Well, young man, we've left you out of the conversation." We'd like to know what you think."

With a perfectly straight face, James told him honestly what was on his mind. He leaned forward and, with better eye contact than he normally exhibits, James said........."I think you're fat!"

Knowing that the doctor deals with autistic children all the time didn't help subdue my twin desires to have the ground open up and swallow me or to laugh hysterically. Fortunately, neither happened.

Nancy Deaves
Toronto, Canada

"Where Do Kids Learn This Stuff?"

While playing minature golf with a group of individuals with autism, one of the group members began to push the golf ball with his club into the hole, rather than hitting the ball. I said to him, somewhat sternly, "You're cheating!"

Without looking up, he said, in a matter-of-fact way, "Men will be men."

Dawn Murphy
Texas

"Fine, Now How About my American Express?"

One day, my husband and I were talking about a friend of ours who was having a hard time with her visa papers and may have to return to her native land. Matthew was very close to this person since she often baby-sat for us. Hearing that she was having trouble with immigration, Matthew "solved" the problem.

"Why don't you just pay her VISA bill so she can stay?"

Sherry and Mitch Anscher
North Carolina

"For Your Ear, Alex?"

Alex has two favorite meals; bacon cheeseburgers and Fettucini Alfredo. He eats reasonably well, but does have limits on the perimeters of his culinary choices. Recently, I asked him if he liked bananas. Obviously giving me a fast answer to shut me up, Alex quickly said, "Yes, I do." So, I prepared cereal with bananas which Alex promptly pushed away with a look of something approaching disgust.

"Alex, you just said that you liked bananas, what's the problem?", I asked in my best semi-patient parent voice.

Alex replied with a logic I wouldn't have dared try on my parents, "I said I like bananas, but I don't like to eat them!"

Jason decided this year that if his six-year-old sister's loose teeth fall out, that his balding father must have "loose hair". Sounds right.

Jean Jasinski
Colorado

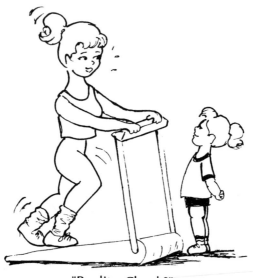

"Reality Check?"

I was happily running on my new treadmill machine. Decked out in the latest slenderizer suit, I was feeling a sense of pride and accomplishment as I turned up the speed to make the belt move faster and faster.

My daughter brought me back to earth as she came in the room and gave her literal interpretation of my efforts.

"My mother....the gerbil."

Diana Daggett
New Mexico

As Alex loves music, I take him to concerts whenever time and finances allow. We've gone to rock star concerts like "Nelson, Paula Abdul, Janet Jackson, etc. However, I also have taken him to the music of Andrew Lloyd Weber, Oklahoma, the Everly Brothers, Wayne Newton, etc. so he gets a real variety.

However, the one he probably enjoyed most was that of Janet Jackson. About four months after the event, as we passed by a newstand, I noticed a headline stating that Ms. Jackson had fallen, was injured and would not be able to perform. I was curious as to how Alex would respond to this sad news and pointed out the headline.

He left me standing there with my mouth open as he read the headline, and walked away saying, "That's okay, Dad, we've already seen her show."

"We Agree with Your Son"

Recently, I took my son to have a check-up. During the process, the nurse rather clinically handed my son a bottle and informed him that she needed to collect a urine sample. He looked confused but did as she asked. Later, as we were leaving, he said, "Mom, you collect vases, and I collect baseball cards. Why does that nurse collect urine?.... Isn't that a funny hobby?"

Lynn Spurgin
Texas

7

"Speak Up!"

Church became a true "experience" with our six-year-old daughter Christina. We would bet beforehand how much of the Mass we would be permitted to attend before our little angel decided she had enough holiness for the day. Most of the time we got halfway through the service.

However, one Sunday was different, or so we thought. She was quiet and pensive. We actually made it through the sermon, which was unusual. At the end, the priest solemnly said, "Let us pray for our intentions" and the Father and the congregation became properly quiet as they prayed. The lengthening silence was more than Christina could stand. Before we could reach our daughter, her voice pealed over the church in a perfect imitation of Sergeant Carter from Gomer Pyle,....

"I CAN"T HEARRRR YOUUU!"

Sometimes we think Christina's only visiting us for our amusement, education and growth.

Tom and Julie D'Amura
Oklahoma

When David was three and a half, my brother, a favorite uncle, came for a visit. In the time he was away, my brother had extensive skin cancer surgery resulting in some gaping wounds on the front and back of his head. For a while, he wore a bandana so as not to upset the children. We all watched David carefully for a reaction when his uncle finally took off the bandana.

David's already big eyes became even wider, but rather than recoil in fear, he got closer to inspected the results of the surgery. With a voice full of innocent awe, he finally whispered to me, "Look, he's broken!"

What a charming and actually appropriate reaction.

(editor's note: Sorry, donor unknown as the wonderful story became separated from the cover letter.)

Alex has a body that any long distance runner would die for; tall and lean, about 80% legs. Partially because of my own background running track and partially stimulated by my desire to have Alex become more physically active, I started taking him out to the local school track. After several outings, I decided to time him in the quarter mile. His first timing set some kind of world record for slowness as he trotted around, flapping his arms, running into people, looking everywhere except in front of him.

I then gave him him a few tips on how to hold his arms, lean into the turns, stride so as to lessen strain, etc. and told him I wanted him to try again and run as fast as he could. After some posturing, he took off and was really running well. I joined him for the last twenty yards encouraging him on as I watched the time. I reveled in his time of I minute and 50 seconds, no world record but a decent time for someone challenged. I congratulated my son, who was leaning over, holding his knees, breathing deeply.

He looked up at me with those baby blue eyes and said, "Dad, why do I have to run so fast just to get back to where I started?"

My son loves riding in the cart at the supermarket, particularly if I give him some candy to enjoy as he rides. One day, I gave him a few Brachs candies that were the seasoned variety. He immediately began spitting them out. I told him that these were the new, "hot" flavors and I had thought he would like them. He responded, "No, I don't want these hot candies; please give me cold candies!"

Lee Werner
Illinois

Ryan was watching "Beauty and the Beast" when the beast turns back into a man. He turned and asked if they now had to rename the movie, "Beauty and the Man!"

Recently Ryan was concerned about breaking the law. He wanted to know who repairs the law when it is broken. Good question.

De Anne Foley
Texas

Alex has fallen in love with playing with words, which has resulted in some very bad puns. (My friends say his tendency to bad jokes is a genetic factor) Here are a few examples, (ed. note: If you have a weak stomach, you may want to skip this part)

"Dad, let's not go to Long John Silvers, let's go to Short Jim Golds!

...

His brother, Justin, was looking for a job in the ads and Alex told him to try the subtracts.

...

He was studying science and he came across the term, 'prey on livestock'. I was concerned that he wouldn't understand such a concept and asked if he knew what that meant. With a smile, he said that the wolves 'prayed' over the animal before they ate it.

...

He went out to dinner with my partner, Polly McGlew, and her husband David. They were kind enough to take him to a very nice German restaurant. When the entrees arrived, he asked what the funny red stuff was on his plate. Polly patiently explained that it was "Rotkohl", a popular dish in Germany. She went one step further, "Rot is German for red, and kohl means cabbage."

Minutes later, David asked what route Polly took to the restaurant, as they had come in different cars. She replied, "I came up Cole street."

Grinning, and without missing a beat, Alex said, "you mean Cabbage Street!"

"The South Will Never Rise Again."

I was showing my stepson some historical pictures in my Virginia home. Naturally, one of my favorites was of one of Virginias' true heroes, General Robert E. Lee. I asked, "Do you know who that is?"

Without any hesitation, but with a somewhat quizzical look, he said,... "Scrooge McDuck?"

Nat Clemon
North Carolina

"There's More Than Way to Make Your Point"

My seven year old son, Christopher, was diagnosed with autism at age two and, although his language is still somewhat stilted, he often communicates well in his own way.

One day he wanted to play with a "magic sword" that was supposed to light up, but did not. He brought it to me for help with a very concerned look, and said, "batteries not included." His resourceful message was understood.

Linda Cavallaro
New York

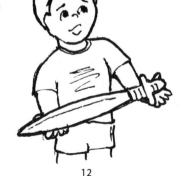

Alex has an Uncle Gary who enjoys him very much and likes teasing him, as he does all the other nieces and nephews. Alex loves the attention. As the family jokester, Gary is usually one-upping other clan members but, intentionally or not, Alex recently got him with this interchange.

"Alex, you sure are good looking, pretty blond hair, big blue eyes, I sure wish I was as good looking as you are." Alex's reply was with a perfectly straight face, "I'm sorry, Uncle Gary, but you're not."

"Is There a Position for This Kid at NIH?"

Matthew has always been concerned with health issues. One of our first experiences was with the soft drink TAB. His father is a cancer specialist and mentioned to Matthew that saccharine had been linked to bladder cancer in rats. He became very upset because I had told him that I'd drank it in my younger days. He seemed reassured when I told him that you had to drink massive amounts to be affected. However, a visit to the supermarket told us that he was still very concerned.

Our son was reading labels on diet soda bottles when an unfortunate soul picked up a six-pack of TAB right in front of him. He launched into an unrequested lecture on the health risks, which he concluded by telling her not to buy TAB because she would get bladder cancer and probably die. The shocked woman did not seem amused in the slightest and I checked out the vegetables as I pretended I didn't know whose child he was.

Matthew also developed a similar perseveration about the health risks of smoking. He would go up to people who were smoking and tell them in a loud voice, " your breath will stink, your teeth will rot, and then you'll die!"

We're not sure there is a future for Matthew as a Senator from our state.

Sherry and Mitch Anscher
North Carolina

"Don't Overcharge Me!"

This year I introduced my nine-year-old son, Matthew, to physical exercise in the form of Tang Soo Do Karate. He takes lessons with a very patient, young instructor, Mr. Peterson, who has encouraged children with disabilities to participate. (Besides autism, Matthew is a below-the-knee amputee.)

One day after class, Mr. Peterson told the students that he was taking orders on karate supplies and mentioned to Matt that he might like a pair of rubber nunchakus. Matt asked, "How much do they cost?" Mr. Peterson said $5.00, as he handed the list to him for review.

Matt seemed a little agitated as he reviewed the product list. Again, he said, "How much does it cost?"

and got the same reply, $5.00. With that response, Matt was more evidently disturbed and again walked away before returning to inform Mr. Peterson angrily that he was wrong!

"It is not $5.00, it is only $4.99!"

Esther Udenberg
Minnesota

My daughter Susan is very high functioning, but still displays definite autistic traits. Recently, she said, in a very serious tone, that everyone with autism should be called, "Autistic Americans". She went on to add, somewhat wistfully, "but they could never unite because they couldn't relate."

Peggy Main
Nevada

Alex talked to his mother after seeing his first professional hockey game.

"Did you have trouble following the puck?"

Pause..."Well, Mom, I wasn't playing."

"The Next Ralph Nader? Lee Iacocca? Henry Ford?"

Eric has a fascination, or perseveration, with automobiles. At four and one-half years of age, he could name virtually every car on the road. How he learned this talent, we're not quite sure. This led to an interesting talk with his therapist.

Trying to test Eric on his ability to recognize things he might see on a daily basis, he showed him a series of pictures and asked Eric if he could identify them. They went through house, t.v., stove, etc. and Eric named them reasonably well. However, when the therapist showed him a picture that he thought would elicit the response, "car", Eric brightened up and said, "Chevrolet Camaro!"

He shocks everyone with this knowledge. One negative is that he expects us to be just as knowledgable and becomes quite upset when we don't have a clue as to the make or model of a car that he can recognize immediately.

Teri Klinger
Ohio

The other day my friend and I were facilitating with my eight-year-old son. I was shocked to suddenly see him type, via the Canon Communicator, some surprisingly strong curse words. I turned to my open-mouthed friend and asked, "Should I wash his hands out with soap?"

From "The Facilitator" Fall 1993 issue

16

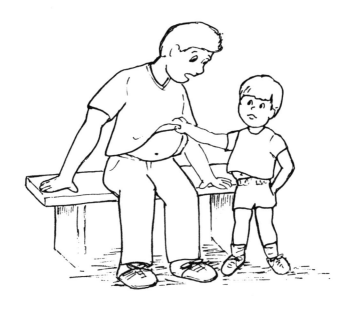

One morning I was helping my nine-year-old non-verbal son get dressed. As I did so, I playfully patted his stomach and told him that he was going to have to start doing push-ups. Without batting an eye, he reached under my shirt and grabbed a big handful of my not-so-lean stomach. His look seemed to say, "I wouldn't talk!"

From "The Facilitator"

My son Buz always greets strangers, with a friendly "Hi!" It's often funny to watch as you can see them trying to remember where they met this friendly young man who just spoke so warmly to them. It gets even funnier when one of the more outgoing strangers answers back, "Well, hello there! How are you doing?"

This puzzles Buz who immediately puzzles the stranger by asking intently, "Do I know you?" It's interesting to watch the reaction.

Sandy Grabman
Oklahoma

TAKING A SHOWER.....THE AUTISTIC WAY

As with most autistic children, our son Mike had his own way of doing things. He especially had a definite pattern to taking his shower. He does much better with written, specific instructions rather than oral. I wrote this several years ago when he was a teenager, and thought you might enjoy it.

1. Go in Bathroom
2. Take shoes into bedroom and put in closet.
3. Back in bathroom, Undress. (For a normal kid, undress would be unnecessary, you might find our kids in the water dressed)
4. Set timer for 15 minutes.
5. Turn on water--be sure both faucets are turned on full force.
6. Get in tub. Wash hair. (Usually, Mike would use five times the normal amount of shampoo.
7. Wash body and wait in tub for timer to ring.
8. Timer goes off. (Normally he would ignore it and stay in the tub until the water was ice cold.)
9. If you hear knock on door, get out of tub.

10. Dry off. Then wrap towel around body and go to bedroom.
(For some reason he would like to spread the towel on floor, perfectly flat and iron out all wrinkles.)
11. Put on pajamas.
12. Pick up towel and take to bathroom, and carefully hang it on towel rack. (He would always do it so that the seams are were perfectly aligned.)
13. Brush teeth and put on deodorant.
14. Back to bedroom and GOODNIGHT!

Monica Moran
Texas

Out into the "Real" World

It is not only necessary but very important that we parents of children with autism venture out into the public. Trips, whether to the grocery store or to another state, become much more "exciting" than with our normal children. We're never quite sure how our special kids are going to perceive an event or how the general public is going to react to our kids. The following stories are about some of those adventures.

Out Into The Real World

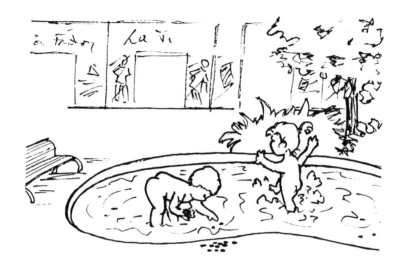

"A Normal Day at the Mall"

At about the age of four, my son became fascinated with pennies and collected them at every opportunity. There was a mall near our home that had a pond that people couldn't resist throwing coins into, mostly pennies. It was almost irrestible for him, so I had to keep a tight rein whenever we were near the pond. However, I did manage to restrain him somewhat with the logic that he couldn't reach in because he might get his clothes wet.

Sometime after I gave him that warning, he and I and his two-year-old sister went to the mall. As luck would have it, my car wouldn't start when we were ready to leave. I put my two children on the bench near the pond and went just a little distance to the phone to call for assistance. I glanced over a few times and they were sitting there quietly and obediently, as I tried to reach relatives or friends who may be able to come to my rescue.

The last phone call must have taken longer than I thought. When I turned around again, they were off the bench, but their clothes were still there. Sans any clothing, they were happily playing in the water, with my son bringing up a treasure of pennies.

Since fluffy towels are not normally included in my purse on trips to the mall, I had to dash into a store to buy something to dry them, while I acted like I had no idea whose children were drawing so much attention.

As I came back out into the mall with my unplanned purchase, I ran smack into a friend from school who lived in another town. After saying hello, she begam laughing about those two cherubs frolicking in the pool with their mother nowhere to be found. In mid-giggle, her eyes dropped down to the towels in my hand and a dawn of understanding crossed her face.

I simply smiled and handed her one of the towels and she willingly helped in my task. As we dried them off, I realized that my son had achieved his goal of getting at those pennies without getting his clothes wet.

Parent
Washington State

"The Case of the 'High-Rolling" Wind Chimes."

To begin, I am an adult autistic individual in my forties. I've gotten over most of my difficulties, but there are, shall we say, some very amusing things that happen along the way that indicate to me my circumstances are life-time, but also that maybe "normal" people share some of my traits more than they think.

Let me explain. During a recent trip to the new gambling mecca of Laughlin, Nevada, I was separated from my party for a few minutes, so I ventured into the hotel's gift shop. Along a windowed wall was row on row of bright silver and gold glittering windchimes. I touched one which began spinning around, glistening as it gave off a monotone sound. This began sucking me in like a vortex. Before five minutes passed, I was playing with all the chimes, fixating on each and every one of them, until a young lady came up to me.

"Aren't they pretty?" she asked. She brought me out of my fixation.

I said, "I guess it looks rather foolish for a grown man to be fondling all this merchandise and making it spin and give off sounds."

"No", she replied. "I think they're pretty. It's nice to meet a sensitive man." Then she changed the subject, "I watched you last night on the roulette table. You were doing spectacular, but you should have quit when you got so far ahead."

I laughed as I said, "Yeah, I ended up donating most of it back."

It was then I realized that my perserverating on the windchimes may have been indicative of my autistic behavior, but my fixation on gambling may be a trait that I share with many.

Fred Beer
California

"Could Make for an Interesting Outing?"

My son tends to focus on several things, but the one that fascinates him the most is women's breasts. It has become such a problem that I literally have to continually tell him, as an endowed woman passes by, "Now,.. mustn't touch,.. mustn't touch."

A few times I've forgotten, which has resulted in making a few friends and a few very irritated strangers.

Janice Abernathy
Ohio

"Guess Who's Coming to Television?"

When Nicholas was eight, he was in the park being watched by his caregiver, Cherie. One minute, he was playing on the swings and the slippery dips. (ed. note: we think slippery dips are sliding boards). The next minute he was gone, running at top speed just disappearing over the horizon as Cherie caught sight of him.   Interestingly, there were three figures on the horizon, not just Nicholas.   As Cherie ran to the last point she sighted him, he was nowhere to be found. The only clue was a wide open door with sounds of a children's program coming out of the house.   She knocked at the door and apprehensively went in when there was no response.

There in the living room was Nicholas, contentedly watching his favorite program as two strange, terrified children sat huddled looking at him, wondering who he was, why he had followed them home and taken over their television set.   They told Cherie that he hadn't said one single word as he followed them out of the playground, kept pace as they ran home and invited himself to their hospitality.

After Cherie gave a brief explanation, the children were calmed and glad they had made a new, but very unusual, friend.

Paul and Coralie Power
Australia

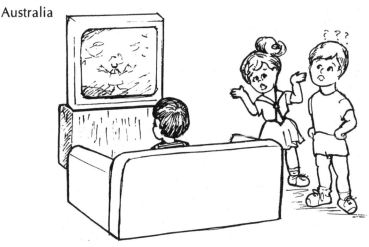

"But You May Have to Wait Five Days"

My husband and I were discussing the best place to buy car insurance when my son offered that we could buy it at the local large hardware store. This puzzled us and we explained that the hardware store didn't sell insurance. He said, "Yes, they do. They sell Smith and Wesson." It took us a few minutes before the bumper sticker came to mind....."Insured by Smith and Wesson."

Parent

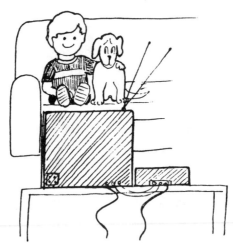

"Be Careful When You Call Your Pet!"

Our four year old son, Caleb, was sent into the basement with his older brother, Zach, to watch T.V. Quickly, there developed a difference of opinion as to which program would be viewed. Caleb had an obsession with "Winnie the Pooh", while my older son wanted his movie. I told Caleb he would just have to wait his turn and left the room. I asked my husband to be the monitor and went about other business. A few minutes later, I checked in to find that my husband was distracted, Caleb was gone, and the front door was wide open.

We began our search aided by other children who sent us in the direction they had seen Caleb run. Shortly, we met a woman who asked if we had lost a little boy. After hearing our relieved, "Yes!", she led us into her home where we found Caleb trying to fit his Winnie the Pooh tape into her VCR. Seems he was petting her dog. When she called her pet, this very surprised lady got two for the call of one as Caleb just trotted in with the dog.

I spoke to Caleb and my not-very-verbal son turned with a look that seemed to say, "I told you I wanted to watch my Winnie!"

Lori Robb
Nevada

"Singing in the shower with your eyes **shut** can save embarrassment!"

Nicholas was enjoying a picnic in the park with his caregiver, Cherie, when he decided to visit one of his biggest obessions, toilets. Off he went with Cherie trying to catch him before he disappeared into the men's bastion. Too late, he disappeared not into the bathroom but into the men's shower.

What was this very attractive young lady to do? Wait and hope everything would be all right or try to go in to insure his safety? She chose to tread where not very many young ladies had ever been and ran into the shower. Almost immediately she stopped dead in her tracks as she came upon a man taking a shower, singing, as he soaped his body and head, **with his eyes closed.**

She was speechless. If she made any noise, what would this man's reaction be? Fortunately, Nicholas suddenly appeared again running right at her. Clamping her hand tightly over his mouth, she grabbed him and quietly led him out of the shower. The cleansing man never knew of the "visitors" and continued happily singing away, shampoo bubbles everywhere, never knowing of his "exposure."

Another fun day, we took Nicholas to a bowling alley where he not only took up the practice of throwing his ball and then chasing it down the alley, but also running **across** the alleys chasing everyone else's too.

Paul and Coralie Power
Australia

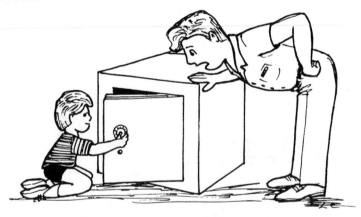

"The First Autistic Willie Sutton?"

When our son was about five, he had exceptional skill with locks. We never knew how he did it but almost any lock could be quickly opened by our small son. One day we took him to the grocery store that happened to have a large safe. It immediately drew his attention. I told my son to get away from the lock However, the clerk intervened to say that it was okay for him to play with it because it was an expensive burglar-proof safe that he couldn't damage, and besides, it would keep him busy while I shopped. Fine with me.

I think I made it through the first aisle before the alarms went off as the huge safe door began to swing open. Both the clerk and the store manager stood there with their mouths open. I'm sure the manager was on the phone immediately to the safe company asking how a five-year-old child could possibly open their burglar proof safe.

Another time, we lost him at the Shriner's Circus. I remembered his fascination as he watched the entryway where the animals came in and out. At that moment, I assumed that he was interested because that was where they were kept. As I began to look for him, I realized, with a rush, that it must have been the lock that had had his attention.

Before I could get to the animal's runway, I found him in the control of some very amazed animal keepers who told me that he had opened the lock to the animal entryway **and** then to the big cat's cage!

Fortunately for everyone, they were sleeping and didn't notice their opportunity for freedom.

Name withheld at parents request

"Many Times They'll Do **Exactly** As You Ask!"

Jeff is never satisfied to just look when we go shopping, a tendency I'm sure he shares with many normal children. Therefore, when we go out, I have to constantly remind him, "touch with your eyes, not your hands." A "normal" child would understand that reproach, even if they don't follow it. Not the case with my Jeff.

While staying at a motel with a beautifully decorated Christmas tree, Jeff was fascinated with the too fragile ornaments. I was afraid that he would break my rule and the expensive tree decorations. That is until I came to the lobby to find that he was following my direction and still enjoying the ornaments. There was my son, pressing his eye delicately against one pretty bulb after the other.

Flo La Roy
Nevada

"Not Your Normal "Day in the Park."

As a teacher of children with autism, I like to expose them to many different environments. One of their favorite outings is to go to the national park. On one of those trips I learned to what extent one of my charges would go to receive his favorite treat.

We were ready to play volleyball when I realized that an important component was missing, the ball. It was there just a moment ago, so one of my darlings had obviously hidden it away somewhere. I encouraged the culprit to bring it back as I spoke to them all about how the entire group couldn't play if we didn't find the ball. No ball appeared. I threatened, gently of course, and even pleaded, all to no avail. Finally, I knew that most of them really liked sweets and I offered a prize for the person who "found" the ball. That got them interested and they all scurried away, looking everywhere.

After ten minutes of searching, there was still no ball, but we were now also missing one camper! We staff members began looking and after a few minutes heard a seemingly far-off voice. We couldn't place it up in the trees or down around the bushes, but we kept following the cries of "help",...."help." We were drawn to one area, but were confused because the cries of help strangely did not seem to come from ground level. As I glanced to my left, I saw a fellow staff member's chin drop as she pointed at, of all places, the outhouse.

We were really glad to find our wayward charge, but not where we did. His voice was not coming from the commode area but from **under** the outhouse. As we held our noses and peered **down** into the commode pit, we saw him up to his hips in undescribable mire, but proudly holding up the volleyball.

After we drew straws to see who would reach down and pull him up, he was rushed (and I mean rushed) to the nearby lake and given a quick bath, while he held on to the volleyball, the key to his prize.

Submitted by a teacher who would rather not be named.

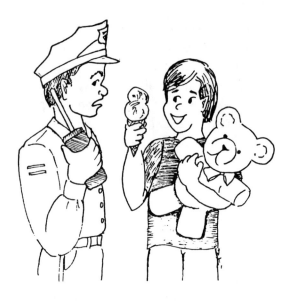

In his book, "Soon will Come the Light", Thomas A. McKean tells of an airline trip where the airline personnel became traumatized by the word autism. Seems that one of his friends casually told the ramp agent that Thomas had autism. Showing a great deal of concern, but an abundance of autism-ignorance, they surrounded this very high functioning author as he began his trip. They checked on him every three minutes for fear he might either try to hijack the plane to parts unknown or physically explode during the flight.

Unfortunately for the flight attendants, there was a stopover, and Thomas had to get off the plane, supposedly in the control of one of the ground personnel. When the agent turned his back to answer another passenger's question, Thomas decided he had enough of this overly protective attention and exited stage left to explore the airport.

When they realized he was missing, they (and we're not making this up) put out an all-points bulletin to find this strange autistic person. However, before they could make the missing persons acquisition of the century, Thomas showed up on his own, after his one-hour traverse of the airport. As he strolled up, eating his ice cream cone and carrying his favorite teddy bear, the security guard grabbed Thomas and screamed into his walkie-talkie, "Target is secure, I repeat, target is secure."

Never having been a "target" before, Thomas tried to make up by offering them some of his ice cream or an opportunity to read his poetry.

Like many young teenagers, autistic or not, Alex sometimes needs to be reminded about common courtesies. This led to my son bringing me up short again. We were about to step into an elevator when two ladies were getting on at the same time. My six foot son almost knocked one down as he barged onto the elevator. I reproached him as I told him he should always let ladies go first on elevators or through doors. He looked confused but said okay.

About one week later, it happened again as we entered a building. He moved ahead of, or should I say through, three women about to go into a large door. I gave him the same admonition. Again, he looked perplexed, so I asked what was bothering him. He said, "Well, Dad, you said that women and men are supposed to be equal. Why do we have to hold doors for them?"

Social Skills

Our friends and loved ones with autism often show their largest gaps of understanding when dealing with social interactions. This gap causes us and the general public consternation and confusion while they blithely go on their way.

This chapter deals primarily with the times we've been set back on our heels by our lovable "bulls in the social china shop."

Social Skills

Alex tries to be considerate of other's feelings, although he shows it in sometimes humorous ways. His efforts in this area led to this conversation after a few "drafted" friends from his junior high school took him to a movie.

> *"Alex, how did you like the show?"*
> *"It was good, Dad."*
> *"Who did you enjoy going to the movies with the most?"*
> *"Dad, I always like being with you best!"*
> *"Well, Alex, that's nice. Thank you." (I felt like a great Dad.)*
> *"Dad, I only said that cause I didn't want to hurt your feelings."*

Alex giveth and Alex taketh away.

"There's Always Hertz..."

As is the problem with most high functioning teenagers with autism, my son does not have the social graces or sensitivity that we would like. This example couldn't have been clearer when one day he was actually asked to go to the school dance by a girl! We were delighted!

However, it was not to be. My less than tactful son said he wanted to go, but his Dad didn't have a car big enough for the girl, who was overweight, to fit into. Needless to say, there was no date.

Parent
Washington State

"Alex May Have a Career Writing Soaps!"

Recently, I was teasing Alex about two of his favorite people, Earl Collins and my partner, Polly McGlew. I told him that they were going to get married (a real legal improbability as Polly is married to David, who Alex also knows). He thought a minute and said, "Oh, they are?"

Realizing that my joke had fallen flat, I added, "They need a place to live. What do you think of them living with us?" This time he thought awhile before answering that he thought that would be okay too. Now I was really getting curious as to his perception of this fictional relationship. "Where would they sleep?"

He pondered only a moment before saying, "Earl can have the Nintendo room (our fourth bedroom where Alex's Nintendo is housed) and Polly can have your bedroom."

"Where will I stay?" I asked trying to look slightly injured. He touched my arm as he said, "That's okay, you can sleep with Polly."

I decided to explain that people that were married to one person were not supposed to marry other people. (I didn't think that it was a good time to explain the Mormon faith, harems or some tribes in Africa.) After briefly explaining the concept of monogamy in marriage, I asked him how he felt about the idea of people being married to only one person at a time.

He looked very serious and said, "if it's okay with you Dad, it's okay with me!"

"What's in a Name?"

The summer that our son, Ryan Foley, turned five, he decided his name should be Norman, his babysitter's husband's name. If someone asked him his name, the answer was always the same...Norman Bickerstaff.

We hoped that the phase would end, but it carried into his first year of school. As he was interviewed by the diagnostician, the interaction was terrific.

"What is your name?"
"Norman Bickerstaff!"
"No, what is your real name?"
"Norman Bickerstaff"
"Your name is Michael Ryan Foley. Now, what is
   your name?"

"Michael Ryan Foley Norman Bickerstaff"

The real Norman decided that he needed to talk to Ryan about being Norman Bickerstaff. He took Ryan into a room and patiently explained that he was the real and only Norman. He returned after quite some time with a triumphant attitude as he proudly instructed Ryan to tell all those assembled his real name. Ryan replied proudly and loudly, "Norman Bickerstaff!"

Looking a little defeated, the real Norman said, "Come on, Ryan, we need to do some more talking!"

DeAnn Foley
Texas

Alex does not have the best sense in the world of social interaction, particularly the often confusing, (even to normal people) world of dating. My efforts to clarify things led to this conversation:

> *"Alex, think you'd like to go out on a date?"*
> *"What's a date?"*
> *"Well, it's where you go to a movie or a play or to the park with someone you like, enjoy being with, and care about."*
> *"Yes, I'd like to do that. Yes, I'd like that!"*
> *"Who do you think you'd like to go with, someone at school?"*
> *"No, ...Earl Collins."*

It was clear that we were on two wave lengths. I was thinking of a few girls that smiled and spoke to Alex

and he was thinking of Earl Collins, who is a nice guy,
but is one of my friends and is 55 years old. However,
when I think about it, Earl did meet the criteria I gave to
Alex as I explained what dating was all about.

"We Hope He Didn't Learn All the Lines..."

My son will watch a movie and pick up on a few lines and repeat them time and time again. Recently, we saw "Pretty Woman" and, for whatever reason, one of the lines stuck in his head. Unfortunately, he didn't leave it there.

I should tell you that my son is in his early twenties, looks very normal, stands over six feet and is a good looking young man.

We went to a fast food restaurant for lunch. It was very crowded with several lines of customers. In the line next to us stood a very nice couple. My son looked at the gentleman who nodded pleasantly and smiled. To my horror, just then the line came out, "That"ll be fifty bucks, mister, and for seventy-five, the wife can watch."

The man's mouth dropped open and you could see the shock and anger in his face. For a second I thought our son was going to be socked in the jaw, but my quick intervention convinced him that it was not personal. However, I noticed that they didn't choose to sit next to us in the restaurant.

Parent

Alex has an interesting perception of family relationships. I asked him how he might like to be an uncle one day. He said that would be okay. His answer felt to me like he might not understand the relationship, so I asked him if he knew how someone became an uncle. He looked puzzled for a moment and then brightened up as he said, "Grow a moustache?"

"Coach "K" Would Love This Kid!"

In an effort to get Matthew more involved with his peers, I encouraged him to follow Atlantic Coast Conference basketball, a near religion in our part of the country. He quickly became focused, or you could say perserverated, on Duke and hated their archrival, The University of North Carolina.

One Christmas, he received a SuperNintendo basketball game in which you can choose names for the two competitors. Naturally, he chose his most and least favorite teams. A typical half-time score was Duke 150 and UNC 0. One day, some adult friends of ours borrowed the game and thought it would be humorous to change all the scores so UNC would appear to be creaming Duke.

After the game was returned, we heard a bellow of dismay from Matthew's room. He came stomping out of his room and told us what had happened. We realized how seriously he took this grievous offense when he said that we should never speak to them again.

He dramatized his feelings by pointing his finger in the air and, using a phrase we assume he heard during the evening news, said, ..."we must sever all ties!"

Fortunately, in time, he forgot his edict and was able to interact with our friends again.

Sherry and Mitch Anscher
North Carolina

One of Alex's less than adept social skills is in introductions. I'm sure it has to do with his inability to understand relationships. Nevertheless, I felt that a little training could help. When we would meet one of his classmates in a mall, or whereever, he would barely acknowledge them, and I might as well as have been a bench as far as Alex introducing me. So, we had our lessons.

The next meeting went like this as we met a classmate, who happens to be Oriental and one of the brightest students in his grade.

"Dad, this is someone from my school." (not great but an improvement)
"This is my Dad." (not bad)

I reached out my hand to meet this gracious young lady as Alex added, "Her name is Ching-Ching Gong---isn't that a silly, funny name, Dad?"

This introduction thing needs more work.

Alex will often explain his feelings in unusual but very succinct ways. He was leaving his mother after a long stay in North Carolina to come back home to Texas. This was their revealing interchange.

"Alex, I'm really going to miss you. I feel sad. Will you miss me?"
"No."
"No? Why is it that you used to cry when you left and now you don't?
"I'm getting used to missing you."

Home

Even in the sanctity and security of our homes, we are subject to the surprises that our special family members can offer. These anecdotes are fairly typical of how even everyday events can turn into "fun" experiences.

Home

"This is a New One on Barney!"

We were beginning to think our son, Andy, would never get toilet trained. We tried potty books, potty videos, thick training pants, treats, and everything anyone suggested.

Finally, merely by chance, we bought Andy underwear with his favorite cartoon characters printed on them. This purchase had an unexpected, beneficial effect.

He started urinating IN THE TOILET, muttering all the while, "Don't pee on Barney...can't pee on Barney."

He wasn't completely trained for a long while, though, as evidenced at a public picnic. Andy announced loud and clear to everyone in the area, "I pooped in Jurassic Park!"

Jayne Kranc
Indiana

"The Miracle Healing.."

Recently, my son, Steven, complained of having a headache. I brought him into the kitchen and put two

Tylenol tablets in his hand. He shook his head and said "No medicine!" I told him he needed to take the pills to make his boo-boo go away. He came up with an answer that he thought would take away his headache without ingesting the life-threatening pills. He simply took the tablets and held them up against his forehead.

Lucie Beauchesne
Massachusetts

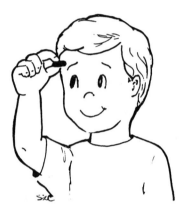

"Just What We Need, Another Disorder"

My "normal" son, Ivan, was taking a bath with our son with autism, Eric. I always felt that that Ivan had minimal understanding of autism, or so I thought. However, during the bath, I heard Eric whining and investigated as to the reason for the unhappiness. Ivan replied, "I keep washing his hair and he doesn't like it."

I asked the obvious question, "Then why are you doing it?" He replied with a smile, "Mom, I can't stop, I have 'washingtism". I loved that.

Michele Viteri
Illinois

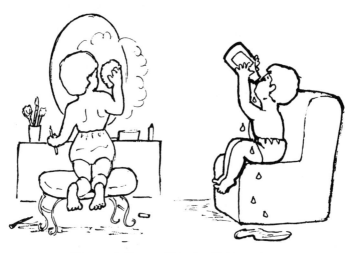

"One of Those "Typical" Days."

I am lucky enough to be the mother of not one, but two sons with autism. To make life even more interesting, they are twins. To put it mildly, things can get pretty hectic. This story may give you some idea.

I answered the phone one day, but couldn't talk to my caller because the noise was so great. So, I went out on the back porch to be able to hear. I glanced into our bedroom and saw Colin bouncing on our bed. He would disappear occasionally and then reappear to continue jumping. In your home, this may have been cause for alarm. In my house, I didn't give it a second thought.

After the conversation, I went into the bedroom to check on him. He was a sight to behold. In the few minutes since I had last seen him, he had opened my makeup drawer, doused the room and himself in white powder and was now standing on his head in the middle of this mess. He saw me and tried to take off.

For once, I was too fast and grabbed him by his powdered head and escorted my white toronado into the shower. With him occupied under the water, I proceeded to vacuum up all the powder.

In the meantime, the other member of my dynamic duo, Patrick, was watching a video. I had hopes that this would keep him occupied while I settled the other problem. I put a "pull-up" on Collin just as the doorbell rang. It was my next-door neighbor, Cheryl, who was bringing some toys for our kids to play with during the summer. As I answered the door, her eyes opened slightly wider as she saw Colin running behind me, completely naked, having relieved himself of his pull-up. I started to explain, but she just shook her head, smiling. Cheryl is a good friend who has seen many unusual happenings at my house and wasn't shocked by this small problem.

After retaping Colin's pants, I went in to check on Patrick. He had decided to have apple juice with his video and was drinking directly from the bottle with about 50% accuracy. Additionally, he had a poopy diaper. What a mess.

After cleaning Patrick up, I felt this ominous sense of quiet, a rare occurence around our house. Colin was nowhere to be found. After a quick, hopeful search of the house, I went for the obvious and looked out the front door. There he was, in the middle of the street, spinning happily in the warm sun. I dashed out to save Colin from being hit by something other than sunrays. He was escorted back into the house and I sat him down alongside a cleaned-up Patrick.

I dropped into the big chair, ready to either cry or laugh. After some consideration, I had a long therapeutic laugh.

Now, only another three hours to lunch!

Susan Egan
Texas

"Home Sweet Home"

Cristina has always been an escape artist. Because of that we worried constantly that she would get out and not be able to get home. Therefore, we taught her our address so that she could at least tell that to strangers.

As she began school, we were comfortable that she had it down pretty well. We didn't know how well.

One day the teacher called to say that Cristina was screaming "7030,.. 7030,.... 7030 now!" They couldn't ascertain what she wanted. Finally, in exasperation, they had called us for a decipherment of this "code." We realized immediately what she wanted. It was our home address.

She just wanted to go home.

Tom and Julie D'Amura
Oklahoma

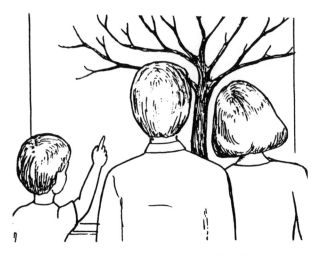

"Can You See What I See?"

As we know, trees lose their leaves in the fall. It's a part of nature that we've seen so often that we take it for granted and miss the wonderment of the change. One fall morning, our son Mitchell came into our bedroom as we had not yet gotten up for the day. He dragged us to the window to show us a "new" sight. We didn't see anything special, but Mitchell did. With all the leaves gone, the large tree in our yard offered something interesting to our son.

"Look, Daddy, it's the V tree!" Sure enough, with all the foilage gone, the tree's branches now formed "V's" all over the tree.

We were again privileged to see the world through Mitchell's eyes.

Jill Gentry
Kentucky

"Happy Birthday, Mom"

A good example of the concrete way my son, Eric thinks, and maybe the way that we avoid things we'd rather not deal with happened at my recent birthday party. Eric has taken to counting ages by saying, "they be four candles old." At my last birthday, I put three candles on my cake. Upon seeing the cake, he said, with some consternation, "Mommy, you not be three candles, you be thirty-two candles!"

Teri Klinger
Ohio

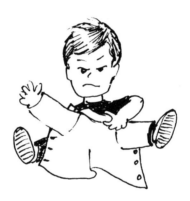

My son, David, has now learned to put his coat on by laying it on the floor upside down, putting his arms in and flipping it over his head. Although, pretty good at it now, at first it was hard for him to get the concept, and we were not as helpful as we could have been. One day, as we were leaving, David began the process but our impatience led us to say, "Hurry up and put your coat on."

So he stopped and began over again, but we saw that this time he was putting it on upside-down.

Again, we repeated the directive, "Hurry up and put your coat on." This time he put his feet in the sleeves. Exasperated, we said, " Your feet don't go in there, hurry up and put your coat on!"

At this point he just stood up, looked at us with disgust and didn't move. It wasn't until we attended a workshop on autism that we understood that if we repeat the same request to David, without proper guidance, he will only assume that he's wrong and will simply begin the process over.

This explained a lot to us. We can only guess what David thought.

Belinda Limbrock
Michigan

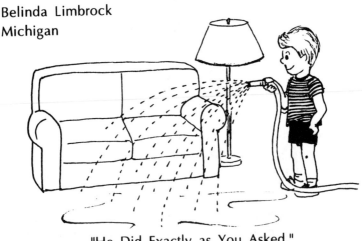

"He Did Exactly as You Asked."

My son, Joseph, loves to play in the water, so seeing him in the backyard with the water hose was not uncommon. One spring afternoon he was in the backyard happily spraying everything he could, when I noticed that it was starting to rain. In my most urgent mother voice, I said, " Come in right now, it's starting to rain." I went on with what I was doing in another room and returned about five minutes later to see if he had, in fact, come in out of the rain.

Well, Joseph had come in, but he had also brought the spraying water hose with him and was smiling as he watered the dining room carpet. I had forgotten to tell him to leave the waterhose outside.

Melanie Kelly
Texas

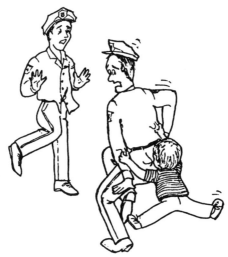

"Is This in the Police Academy Handbook?"

My son, Jacob, is now a well behaved ten-year-old and mild mannered, but at the age of five he was nothing of the sort.

One day I came home to find that our home had been burglarized. I waited for the police, holding onto Jacob, who did not want to be held because he wanted to go run in the back yard. When the police arrived, I brought (or rather pulled) Jacob into the house so I could speak to the officers. I tried to answer questions as I wrestled with my son. The officers were somewhat bemused at my difficulty with this small child, but went on with their report. Suddenly, Jacob left me and, before anyone could move, lunged at one of the officers and bit him in the stomach. Far worse, he didn't let go!

The policeman, who minutes before was wondering why I couldn't control that innocent little kid, was now yelling, "get him off of me!" I got Jacob by one leg and the other officer grabbed the other as we tried to shake him loose. The cop was screaming his head off, dancing around the room with my child attached to his abdomen and two adults attached to the child. I'm yelling, "Don't hurt him, he doesn't understand!" (I didn't feel that this was the time for an indepth explanation of autism, or an update on his latest A.R.D., or the joys of behavior modification).

When Jacob decided to let go, the officer had a torn shirt and was bleeding slightly. The other officer suddenly realized that he might be the next target and turned to run....but not fast enough. Jacob got him too, a direct hit on the right buttock. As we were prying him loose, I wondered how he was going to explain the marks to his wife.

Both officers, now out of imminent danger, hastily left the house. One yelled over his shoulder, "You can come down to the station house to file your report, but for God's sake, don't bring him!"

Linda Todd
Texas

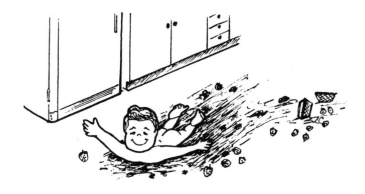

"Sounds Like Fun to Us!"

Jeff enjoys sensory stimulation, and we frequently find him sandwiched between the bare mattress and the fitted bedding or underneath a heap of pillows. He enjoys the feeling of rubbing fabric against his stomach and bare chest. Jeff also likes strawberries both to eat and to feel.

Recently, I came in from being out for the evening and heard a strange, funny story from my husband, verified by strawberry remains. Jeff had obviously taken a basket of strawberries and had smashed them on the kitchen floor. Hearing giggles and sounds of delight, Dad decided to investigate.

The scene was one we'll never forget. Dad saw his son, happily and with a big smile, sliding across the "lubricated" floor on his bare stomach in crushed strawberries. Who knows what Jeff was thinking, but he was obviously enjoying his "landing strip" very much.

Flo La Roy
Nevada

My husband and I returned home from a vacation to find most of our family obviously happy to see us as they excitedly said, "We missed you." and "I'm glad to see you." Our son with autism remained aloof and quite silent. This was not uncommon and we were not bothered by the lack of response to our return.

However, at dinner the truth came out in an unusual way. After eating, he folded his hands behind his head, leaned way back in the chair and exclaimed, "It's good to be home." We knew what he meant and it felt just as good as the other responses.

Parent
Washington State

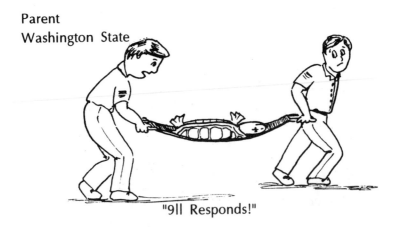

"9ll Responds!"

When my son was younger, he had a pet turtle named David. One day, his pet burrowed under our neighbor's fence and unfortunately was attacked by their dog. David was retrieved but with damage to his undercollar. He subsequently became sick. I tried to resuscitate him by taking him to the bathroom and placing him in water.

The next thing we knew there was an ambulance on the way to our door. This was the message 911 received from our son, "My mother is in the bathroom with David, who was hurt by the dog and may be dying... there are bubbles coming out of his mouth and we need an ambulance right now!"

He omitted mentioning that David was a turtle.

Fortunately, the dispatcher was understanding (we think) and the ambulance was recalled.

Parent
Washington State

"The Power of Advertising"

At an early age, our son wanted very much to purchase tampons. The reason?... because he remembered the ad that said, "with tampons you can do anything!"

When he first went out on his own, I worked with him on planning and preparing his own meals. For a period of time, I offered to fix dinner, but breakfast and lunch were up to him. So off he went shopping. Shortly, he returned home and proudly displayed his purchases, a large can of Ultra Slimfast, a quart of milk and tampons. I already knew why he bought the tampons, but his reasoning for the diet meal was a little confusing until he reminded me of their ad, "a delicious meal for breakfast or lunch"

Name withheld at parents request

"There's More Than One Way to Clean Up!"

Our family Saturday project was to scrub oil spills off the driveway. I'd just gotten started when I had to go back inside for another bucket of water. When I returned, I found my son, who has autism, scrubbing merrily away while he was holding his face close to the stain and yelling at the top of his lungs. At first I was totally confused, until I noticed the detergent we were using, "Shout." You've guessed it, he was following their slogan and was trying to "Shout it out!"

A Parent

Here's a letter to a mother that is priceless, maybe in more ways than one.

Dear mom,
I have been very good this year.
For Hanukkah I would like:
Nuts, Pecans, a Toy....and a Rolex.
Love.
Adam

From the "Facilitator"

The Workplace

More and more, thankfully, young men and women with autism are being introduced to the workplace. The combination of our young people with the propriety of the business world can cause some very humorous situations.

The Workplace

"When Dealing with Time, Be Precise!"

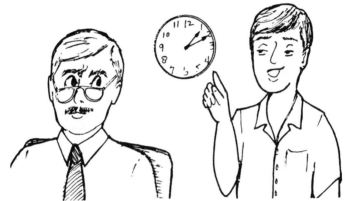

My son got his first job in the real world in his mid-twenties. We were all pleased that he was able to adapt, and the employees were accepting of his less than normal work habits, such as refusing to lick or even wet envelopes to close them but instead sealing them all with packing tape. One day, the boss of his supervisor came in and turned out the overhead light that flooded both his office and the area where Mike was working. He quickly turned on a lamp so Mike could work and told him that it would only be about five minutes and that he needed the light off to see a computer screen in his office.

The big Boss went on reviewing the screen in his office while he answered the phone and handled interruptions. Finally, with all of that out of the way, he turned to the screen in the darkened room, only to have the office suddenly completely light up.

He swirled to chastise the offender who had turned on the light, only to see Mike pointing to his watch and saying, "Five minutes, your time is up!"

Anita Ferman
Texas

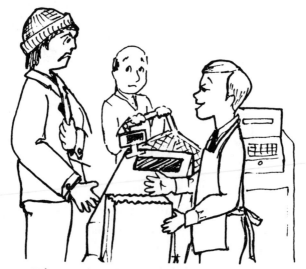
"The Perfect Supermarket Detective."

My son was in a job training program that took him to a local grocery store. He had several of the jobs there, one of which was as the cashier. Once he learned the function he was really pretty decent at the job. However, his seeing the world exactly as it is led to an interesting situation.

He was checking out one customer, who obviously didn't value honesty very highly. He tried a trick that other petty thieves have pulled off easily on young people working the cash register. However, he hadn't run into anyone like my son. As he neared the counter, he put two items on the moving belt and another two under his jacket.

My son hardly even glanced at him as he rang up not two but four items. The customer complained about the "overcharge." The "cashier from autism", matter of factly, informed him that he rang up the two items he was hiding under his coat. Our would-be thief exited as rapidly as possible.

We found this interesting because our son appears so unaware, yet he is often acutely aware, even when he gives the impression that he doesn't have a clue.

Parents name withheld at their request

"Mr. Bumble's Advice"

I made the tough decision to give up my job as an editor to devote my time and energies to our daughter, with autism, Maureen. Obviously, I had to tell my boss, Mr. Bumble. This is a gentleman who, at least within his own mind, is a legend in the media world.
He was definitely also the kind of man who doesn't like losing. It was certain that he would not like losing his editor, right-hand man and heir-apparent.

I went into great depth as I explained about Maureen and how she needed non-stop, minute-to-minute attention from someone with a tremendous of energy and strength. Someone who could work with her endlessly----hour after hour---with a truckload of patience.

At first he seemed to understand, as he nodded his head and seemed deep in thought. However, I soon realized that the thought process was not one of sympathy but of seeking inventive ways to keep me. I could work at night, on the commuter train, when she slept, when I slept, etc. Mr. Bumble's ideas were definitely getting weird. I tried hard to stay flexible but, clearly, my days on his magazine were over. Still, he kept talking and I kept giving the same answers and the same reasons explaining time and again how difficult and time demanding this challenge was going to be..

Finally, after he had just about ground me down to a fine white powder, he gave in (or so I thought) and admitted that I would have to look after Maureen full-time. Then, he gazed off into space for a long time and then turned back to me and said, (I swear this is true) "Well, you know, Joe, it doesn't have to be all bad. I mean, maybe you could do something productive with all that free time, and write a book or something!"

Joe McKeon

In the last book, I mentioned that children with autism are certainly more honest and upfront that the general population and when they do lie, they are very transparent at it. This story illustrates that point as the examples did in the first book.

My adult son with autism works at the Eton center and is generally good about going in to his job. However, one day he was reluctant, so I asked his supervisor at the center to talk to him. This was their conversation, as I handed my son the phone.

"Why aren't you coming in?"
"Can't, my mother's been robbed and raped by burglars."
"I just spoke to your mother."
"No, I'm telling the truth, she's lying at my feet,.......dead!"
"Can I speak to your mother?"
"No, she's calling the fireman because our house is on fire and is burning down."

After some conversation, the case worker made it clear that he wasn't going to buy into these stories.

"What is the real reason you can't come into work?"
"I just don't want to."
"Well, how would you like to come on in, and we'll have lunch and talk about this?"
"Oh, that sounds nice, I'll be there."

Sandra Davidson
New Jersey

"Did You Hear the One About...?"

I often have the responsibility of going out to speak to those in the general community, particularly as it relates to placing some of our clients in jobs.

Recently, I went to a factory in an area of Trenton that is predominantly Polish. I launched into my explanation of autism and emphasized that they had to be concrete in their directions. That they should say "move faster" if they wanted our client to increase speed. I warned that an urging of "move it along" could find everything on the desk on the floor or some other "interesting" interpretation.

One lady, who was a supervisor, raised her hand and offered an anology that caught me way off guard. "So, it's just like being Polish!" My mind searched wildly for her meaning. Was I about to be hit with a Polish joke in this environment? Did she totally misunderstand my explanations?

Finally, after what seemed an eternity, she added, "You see, a lot of these people don't speak very much English so, I have to be very clear and it always works better if I show them what to do, rather than tell them."

I doubt if this woman had very much formal training in behavior management or education but she certainly taught me something that day. Now, I talk about visual cues in all my presentations.

Peter Gerhardt
New Jersey

School

Tuning our children loose in an educational atmosphere offers untold opportunities for laughter. The structures required in a school are usually fine with our kids as long as they meet the guidelines of what our children, in their unique way, consider to be sensible. When they don't meet that test, look out! You'll all enjoy these, but if you're a teacher or educational professional, you're really going to love the following.

School

"Our "Letterman?"

I was teaching my son letters, trying to instruct him in hearing the first letter of a word, as that would help him to sound it out. I felt like I was getting nowhere fast. Finally, I thought I had the perfect key. His name is Warren Werner, so I said, "Listen, your name is Warren Werner. What is the first letter of each?

He brightened up as he gave the literal and correct answer to my question,...."E."

Lee Werner
Illinois

"Say What?"

My favorite stories are the ones that show that my son, Ted, understands more, **much more,** than he's given credit for. In fact, I rejoice every time he outsmarts me. This happens more often than one might expect, often unpredictably.

Recently, Ted and I had a discussion about his younger brother who is a student at the University of

Washington. I explained that he took science classes. Receiving a blank look, I assumed a lack of understanding and asked, "Ted, do you know what 'science' means?"

"No", he answered.

Groping to define the word, I began; "Well, 'science' means 'study' or 'knowledge'. So, a scientist is a person who knows a lot about a certain area. For example, there are scientists who study different forms of life. They are called 'biologists."

When his eyes still looked blank, with no apparent glimmer of recognition and very little interest, I tried an example that might mean more to Ted. "There's a name for all scientists. For an example, there's even a name for people who study animals. They are called 'zoologists.'"

Still trying to communicate my wisdom to my son with the sphinx-like smile, I added, "There's even a word for people who study reptiles." I tried to think of the term, couldn't, and looked for another example. "There's a special name for scientists who study fish, too." Again, I, the teacher couldn't come up with it.

Ted noticed my cause in concentration. As I tried to remember the difficult word, he leaned forward and gave me another lesson in underestimating Ted, "Do you mean an "ichthyologist?"

Charley Hart
Washington State

"Words to Live By"

On the way home from school one day, my three boys, including my son with autism, Jeremy, were discussing what they had learned in school that day. My oldest said, "Just say no to drugs." The youngest piped up with another important rule, "Never get into a car with a stranger."

I asked Jeremy if he knew of any important rules. He responded with, "Never call a girl stupid."

I found out later from Jeremy's teacher that he had gotten into a lot of hot water before he learned this particular rule.

Bonita Gallen
Texas

"A New Twist on the Old Testament"

We try to mainstream our son into society at every opportunity. This desire led us to having Ted attend Sunday School. It didn't seem to be going too well. We would ask him simple questions about the lesson and there would be no response. So, I decided to sit in on the class with him and ask him questions immediately after class.

That Sunday, the lesson was a film about Abraham and Isaac. As the plot unfolded, Abraham took his beloved son up to the mountain to be sacrificed as commanded by God. I began to worry. "What have I done to this child, forcing him to watch something he's bound to misunderstand?"

It got worse. After Isaac got a reprieve, Abraham slaughtered a ram caught by the horns in a bush. Then Sarah's jealousy of the slave woman and her son caused her to insist that Abraham banish them both to the desert forever. Mercifully, the movie stopped and I turned to Ted reluctantly and asked "What was the movie about?"

Ted turned his head and uttered a single word, one-word summary,.... "Cannibals."

With all apologies to theologians, we believe that if one had to reduce that complicated storyline to a succinct term, "Cannibals" would be hard to beat.

Charley Hart
Washington

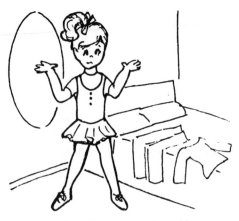

"Mother's Need to be More Specific..."

My daughter is pretty good at getting ready for school. I would lay out her clothes and she would follow my directions. Recently, it got even better as she would pick out her clothes and get ready, usually with some prompting from me. However, this improvement led to an interesting problem.

About three weeks into her independence, she came home from school appearing very unhappy. I inquired as to why the long face. She almost cried as she related how she wore a dress every day and the other kids got to wear pants and shorts. I was shocked.

"Darling, you have all kinds of other clothes, why don't you wear those?' I said. She looked as shocked at my statement as I had hers. "Mother, it's your fault, every morning you tell me to go in and get **dressed.**"

Virginia Unverzagt
Illinois

Alex has become a very social young man, although his friendliness takes on an open, charming, but by our "normal" standards, inappropriate manner. He'll talk to anyone relaxed and without embarrassment..

Recently, a new teacher (not teaching one of Alex's classes) came to his junior high school . Between classes, she assumed her place in the hall observing student traffic. She was surprised to have this tall young man come up to her, put out his hand and said, "Hello, I'm Alex Gilpin. You're new here and I've never met you and you've never met me, so now you know who I am."

I'm reasonably certain that this was the only introduction like this that she received. However, this is one instance where Alex may have been the truly appropriate one.

High functioning children with autism will often write letters that must be surprising, at the very least, to the outside world. The following correspondence from a young man to his teacher and the principal of his school after taking a bus trip illustrates this point.

DEAR MRS. MORRIS AND MRS. KOWNACKI,

THANK YOU VERY MUCH FOR INCLUDING ME IN YOUR FIELD TRIP TODAY. I LIKED TAUM MOUNTAIN STATE PARK.

LOVE, JEFFREY

PS. THANK YOU FOR LETTING ME RIDE RYDER BUS 289. I LIKE GREEN SEATS BETTER SO NEXT TIME SEE IF YOU CAN GET A BUS WITH GREEN SEATS.

Sandy Kownacki
Missouri

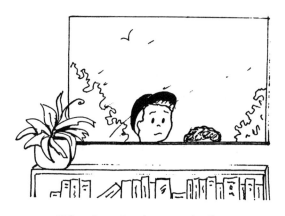

"The Boy in the Baseball Cap."

There's a boy out front in a baseball cap, staring in my window...

When our son, Tommy, was young, he was a "runner," When we'd park the car at the mall, before we could get out of our seatbelts, he would be out of the back door, running down the traffic lane toward the mall entrance door. He loves the beach, so anytime we stopped our car anywhere near the surf, he would be out like a little jet, running toward the water, all three-foot- six of him, with hands waving and shoelaces flying. This might sound harmless, but we had to stop in traffic once, unfortunately in sight of the beach. He was gone.

As he grew older, although he's had his challenges and with his behavior somewhat undependable, he is capable of the curriculum at his school and is a manageable young man.

Recently, he showed that he was more capable than we might have thought. He rides the handicapped bus. One of the other children is Fashid, a nine-year old who loves to dash off, as Tommy did in his early years. Tommy was given the responsibility of holding tightly to Fashid's hand and guiding him from the van to the school. Tommy accepted the responsibility well.

One day, there was a substiitute driver, who made a simple error when arriving at the school building. There were two entrances, and the driver let them out at the front door, not the rear. Our sons stepped off without protest. This could have been serious trouble.

However, Tommy took firm control of Fashid and took action that was effective, if not appropriate. He walked his charge the 50 feet to the school office window. Without saying a word, he simply stood there, in the shrubbery, with Fashid's hand tightly held in his. So, for about ten minutes, he just stood there, looking in the window, baseball cap slightly askance, with a very serious look on his face.

The secretary of the autistic program, realizing that they were late, called down to the main office to see if anyone had seen the missing kids. Her question was what caused the school secretary to say,....

"Well, yes,..... there is a boy in a baseball cap who is staring in my window."

All's well that ends well.

Harry Richards
Pennsylvania

"If God **really** wanted me to learn the Torah...."

On Thursdays, I pick up Matthew from school to take him to Hebrew class. One particular day, we were experiencing some pretty fierce storms, with violent lightning and thunder. Matthew has always been more than a little unnerved by thunderstorms, so **he** decided we should go straight home and skip Hebrew class. I reassured him that it would be safe, but he didn't seem particularly relieved.

When we got to his teacher's home, he refused to get out of the car. I tried to urge him, but to no avail. Then his teacher came out of the house and said it was important to have the class and to come on in.

Matthew not only refused but made his feelings very clear when he rolled the window down and yelled, "I will not risk my life for Hebrew!"

Sherry Ansher
North Carolina

Alex was studying history and, as that was my major in college, I was meddling or helping (take your pick). We came upon the term "Alien and Sedition Act."

Now, Alex does learn historical terms, but his understanding of the concepts is very limited. Therefore, I asked him if he knew what that act did. He had no clue. So, I explained that it was intended to keep a certain group of people out of the country. I asked him if he knew who they were.

"Lawyers?".... was his instant reply.

Alex's idea would have probably been a lot more popular.

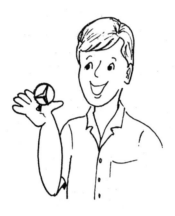

"At Least He 'Borrows' Quality."

Shortly after graduating from high school, our son got his driver's license. One of his first trips out was to apply for a job. He returned home, very happy and excited. We assumed that the interview went well, but that was not the reason for his happiness. He had a new acquisition. Unfortunately, he had taken the hood ornament from a new Mercedes-Benz that was parked near his car. We were reasonably sure that the owner was not aware of our son's acquisition.

We were shocked that he would do such a thing in the first place, but then that he would tell us, and with pride! When asked, he said that it made him feel normal. Why? It turns out that many of his fellow students at school had "collections" of hood ornaments that they had taken. So he thought that if he took the ornament it would help him to be more like them.

Sometimes, I'd rather he didn't emulate "normal kids."

P.S. We went back to the Mercedes, left a note and our "innocent" son paid for it from his first week's pay.

Parent's name withheld at her request

"When Will They Learn?"

My son was placed in with regular students, without the teacher being informed of his limitations. This led her to ask him to leave class because he was doing "Rainman" imitations.

Name withheld at parent's request

I've always been a big proponent of inclusion, whenever humanly possible. When Alex was in a preschool group, however, he was in a "special" room with children of all handicaps. One day, I noticed my not very verbal son limping badly. The movement led me to check his shoes for a stone. No stone, no wound of any kind, no tenderness, no indication that he had any kind of pain. I was really confused until the next morning when I took him to school and saw one of his classmates who had polio. Alex had copied the child's limp perfectly.

I used this story in the next ARD to demonstrate how Alex could learn and emulate his classmates. I said, "If he can learn this movement so perfectly, just by observing, than he can certainly learn behavior from normal children."

That argument helped to carry the day to have Alex join the first grade class.

Poignant

As I mentioned earlier, the first "Laughing and Loving with Autism" had a concluding chapter called "poignant." Although not planned at the conception of the book, it was very popular and we have more wonderful and touching stories to share with you.

These stories are from parents, siblings and those with autism. If you read them carefully and maybe for a second time, you will see that, in many ways, they are as much about the writer as they are about the subject.

Poignant

You just found out your child has autism?

It's not all that bad, folks!

Sure, having an autistic child in the family does cause some problems and the parents must change a lot of their preconceived notions of childrearing. But that's not necessarily bad.

For instance, our son, Buz, has needed many years of speech therapy, special education, summer camps and fourteen months of hospitalization. However, I feel that this "challenge" has given us an advantage other parents don't have. These teachers, therapists, and doctors have been the most caring, nurturing people we've ever known. With generations of families so widely scattered these days, how many parents have the benefit of such support.?

Buz has helped us to get to know the people in the neighborhood, indeed in the entire city. He was always innocently curious. Buz would go up to strangers and ask all about the supermarkets in their areas or pipe organs in their churches. They would quickly realize that they were dealing with a very lovable, although, granted, unusual person.

Once people get to know him, they like him very much and feel somewhat protective of him. It's not uncommon for me to meet people for the first time who live many miles from my home, who break out in a smile and say, "Oh, you're Buzzy's Mother!" He just seems to bring out the best in people. He has made all of our lives better and more fulfilling.

Sometimes I feel sorry for families with only "regular" kids. Their lives must be so boring!

Sandy Grabman
Oklahoma

"Sometimes We Wonder Just How Much They Do Understand!"

The first step in my plan to get back into shape was to join an aerobics class. This was a new venture for me, having never before joined an organized exercise class. All of my previous efforts had been personal and individual.

The first class was a personal disaster. Not only was I out of breath trying to keep up with the others who were in better shape (and mostly younger), but I was also having trouble following the instructions quickly.

My son, James, who has autism, was there as I explained to my normal daughter, Jennifer, how her mother had embarrassed the family name that day. I laughed as I explained how when they were up, I was down, when they were moving forward I was moving

back and I was always always one beat off. She was delighting in my story and we weren't sure James was even listening. However, he obviously was as he surprised us both by speaking up and saying,
"Yeah, Mom, it was just like autism, huh?"

I was too shocked at his perception then to respond, but yes, James, I suppose what I experienced was how you see the world.

Nancy Deaves
Ontario, Canada

My son Jeremy's teacher is very good at saving special papers for me that he does in class. Since he generally throws all his schoolwork and notes from the teacher away before he gets home, this is a very good idea. One paper that I will treasure forever was a writing assignment he had to do about someone important to him. It was particularly significant because I don't often hear these thoughts.

"My mother is a teacher at Miss Jewell Elementery. (sic) My mother's also a great mother. She loves me much. I like her even if she gets mad at me. I love her."

Bonita Gallen
Texas

Alex stays with his mother during the summer and enjoys it very much. This summer she arranged for him to have voice lessons. He seems pretty happy about it as he loves almost any contact with music. She arrived to pick him up after the lesson and arrived a little early. Not wanting to embarrass him, she waited in the hall.

From there she could hear him, but he couldn't see her. She stood there with tears running down her face as she listened. It wasn't at the fact that he was doing so well, but it was the song his nice voice was singing out. Her son with autism, for whom there had been so many, many gloomy predictions, was singing, ..."You'll Never Walk Alone."

The following was written by an nine-year-old boy about his feelings for his brother.

"My Brother. David."

I don't think people should make fun of handicapped people because they are different, in different ways. I don't think autistic people are mean or bad, they are just different from us. They were born that way.

My brother is handicapped. I don't like it because my brother can't play football with me, because he does not understand. I told him to make a touchdown, but he just stood there. I had to show him what to do. If I tell my brother to do something, he will yell at me and I get scared. One time, when we were playing with toys, and my friend was over, we went upstairs. David was playing Jurassic Park. I asked David if he would play with me and my friend. He got mad and threw toys at us.

My brother goes to a special class with other handicapped kids. I feel sorry that he is autistic, but I'm still lucky to have a brother. I don't like it when he imitates me, but that's how he learns things from me. I would be alone if he was not here, and I wouldn't have anyone to play with very often.

I know he is not like people are used to, but I love him. Even is he is not like everybody else.

Dale Limbrock
Michigan

"He's Still David."

When you have a handicapped child, there are a lot of times that people make cruel comments or say things that they think will help but are inappropriate.

There are, however, those occasions that someone says something that does help, and will stay with you for a lifetime. One such comment came from my father the day we told him that his grandson was handicapped.

That day, as my husband and I were sitting with my parents at their kitchen table, I was very nervous. I wasn't sure how they would take the news. We said that we had something important to tell them about David. When we told them he was autistic and mentally handicapped, I started to cry. I looked at my mother, and could see the tears beginning to form in her eyes. I looked at my father, and he looked up at us and said firmly, "He's still our grandson, he's still our David."

At that moment, I knew that he was right. Nothing had really changed. He was still David. He was still the same little boy we loved so much. David is fortunate to have grandparents who love him for **who he** is, without qualifications.

Brenda Limbrock
Michigan

Ed. note: We feel that, in many ways, David Limbrock is a very lucky boy.

"The Language of Love"

My son, Micah, has autism. Though he is verbal, his speech is limited. He has come a long way in the past few years, but there was a time when I wondered if Micah would ever use meaningful language to communicate. I wanted so much for him to tell me his favorite color, what was behind his fascination with stop signs or what he wanted for Christmas. Anything spontaneous would have been appreciated. Most of all, I wanted to hear him say to his mama ..."I love you."

One wonderful day, I rented the Walt Disney movie, **Beauty and the Beast.** Micah loved it, especially the music. When the movie was over and the credits began to roll, I got up to leave the room. Micah stopped me and took hold of my hands. At first, I thought he was afraid I was going to turn off the tape before the credits were finished, (An unforgiveable crime to Micah's way of thinking).

However, I was surprised when Micah looked up at me and, in his own language, asked me to dance. As the credits rolled and the theme played, my son layed his head against me and slowly began to sway. When the song was over, he stopped "dancing", looked me straight in the eye and said, "I love you, Mama." The words were soft and a bit slurred, but they were unmistakeably genuine.

It's been two years since Micah first spoke his words of love. I am still moved every time I recall his gift. As he continues to grow and learn, I find myself taken with the way Micah makes up with me after we have had some kind of disagreement. When all is said and done, Micah brings the situation to a close by saying, "I still love you, Mama."

Beverly Phillips
South Dakota

Alex had unique ways of showing affection when he was younger. There was one lady that I could tell he liked, but he didn't show the caring until one interesting afternoon. He approached my friend, turned his back to her, took her hand over his shoulder and held it to his chest.

We often say that our siblings gain from having a challenged sister or brother. This story illustrates that point.

My daughter Rachel asked why God gave Michael autism. I replied that I didn't know exactly but I was sure that some good would come out of it and that we would all be better for having to help him.

Shortly after that conversation, her teacher told me how compassionate and patient Rachel was in class. She related how Rachel was particularly tolerant of a fellow student who is speech delayed and often pinches and pokes to get attention. Rachel continues to befriend him despite all of that and is very helpful. I suppose I answered Rachels question appropriately and her quality has shown through.

from the "Facilitator"

"First Words."

All parents await the first words their child will speak. Not knowing that we were dealing with an autistic child, we had just assumed we had an "eccentric" on our hands. The language was delayed, but the "experts" told us to wait and not to worry.

When we did notice new words, they were always nouns and never verbs. She would sing hymns from church but never would construct sentences. We were perplexed. The most confusing incident came when we discovered our daughter's memory abilities, but were not yet aware that we were dealing with autism.

The events of that afternoon had me thinking for a brief moment that everything was okay. In reality, I was being introduced to one of the phenomena of strange disorder.

I was watching television after a hard day at work. I was relaxing and only half-awake. Cristina came to me with a look of puzzlement on her face. I was aware that she was there but was startled to hear her speak in clear English and with correct grammar and syntax. Clearly, I heard her. She said, "Daddy, I don't understand." At first, I thought I was asleep and was dreaming or hearing the T.V. I sat upright and said, "What don't you understand, honey?"

I was astonished to be speaking to Cristina. She looked me straight in the eye and repeated the question. Again, I answered and again the same question. I was beginning to feel delusional. I was having a conversation of sorts with someone who had never spoken before. I ran upstairs to get my wife ro find out what was going on.

My wife had already experienced something similar to what I had just gone through. It took us a while to figure out what was going on. It was a function of this strange disability that we would come to know very well. The daddy Cristina was referring to was King Trident from the movie "The Little Mermaid" and the line was one delivered by his daughter. We later learned that she had memorized various lines from all the Disney movies. Eventually, she got to the point she could recite almost complete scripts.

My afternoon and our interactions with Cristina would have been much clearer if we only we had known sooner that we were dealing with autism.

Tom and Julie D'Amura
Oklahoma

Sadly, some educational professionals appear to be part of the problem to parents, not a part of the cure. This poem offers some insight to that feeling.

I'll play your game if I have to
But I don't like it
Chess is okay
But not when I'm one of the pieces
And my child is only a pawn

Paula Maziar
California

"Martine at Three"

I remember you standing
On your slide
Not sliding, just standing
Waiting.
Your head held high,
Nose to the wind.
Like a deer
Watching

For hours it seemed
You did not stir
Except for your hands
Flapping
I look at you and wonder,
Why are you this way?
What do you seek by
Listening?

I heard a voice
In my heart cry out
God help her
Thrive.
I feel so helpless
Watching you struggle
With your handicap
Autism

Yet, I am in awe
Of your innocent faith

And childlike trust
Hoping
That someday the world
Will not frighten and confuse
Until then you stand on your slide
Waiting

My daughter, Martine has come a long way since I
wrote this poem. I celebrate her courage and the
determination of all who have worked with her
especially my wife, Patty.

Chuck Munier
Maine

Empty Noises

Looking at you
Looking somewhere else
In McDonalds.

Happy meals and fries
Don't fill the empty silence
Amid the chaos.

The constant chatter
Of other 3 and 4 year olds
Surrounds you and I.

In the car
On the way home
I ask
"Was your cheeseburger good?"

In the rear view,
I notice a mother and son
(who are about the same age as you and I)
Talking back and forth in the front seat.

Their conversation seems to never end
As we wait for the light to turn green
In our silence.

Connie Post
California

"A Sister's Love"

In my profession as an autism consultant, I met
this delightful young lady who has an older brother
with autism. My conversations with her took the
normal range of ups and downs but also evidenced her
strength as she said that anyone who could not accept
her brother wasn't a friend anyway.

However, she helped me to realize that a sibling
doesn't merely deal with what is there but also deals
with what she is missing, particularly in an older
brother. The confidant, protector, mentor factors that a
younger sister hopes to feel from an older brother
simply can't be realized... Still, she spoke of hope and
love. Her poem that follows was one I found very
touching.

Cindy Waddell
Oregon

"Brother"

What goes on behind your eyes
In your mind?
I want to know
Are you real?
Sometimes, I'll see a glimmer
And maybe I'll hope
But I get afraid..
And crawl back into my shell....just like you
There are things I want to say to you
And do for you
Because you're my brother
Aren't you?
You have your walls
And I have mine.
Do I try hard enough to break your walls down?
How hard should I try?
Could you even tell me...
Or do I have to be strong by myself?
One day your walls will come down
Your shell will break open,
And I'll find a way to say to you...
Hello.....I am your sister...You are my Brother
And I've always loved you.

Donnie

*Alex and I were sharing some cookies. I started playing with him, as I told him to look at that monster "over there," and when he did, I would take one of his cookies. Quickly, he caught on, or so I thought, and was enjoying the game. Then, to my delight, he told me to look away. When I did, with a smile, he reached up and grabbed one of **his** cookies and hid it.*

As the Mind Dismisses, the Heart Embraces."

I understand that my offering in the first
"Laughing and Loving with Autism," was appreciated by
those who read it and identified with the dreams of
many of us who love a child or adult with autism.
I was asked by my father to donate another writing to
this book. As I am privileged to have Alex as my
brother, I'm also delighted to share my loving, but
unscientific views on autism.

All of us who live with autism live with an
incomprehensible duality. On one hand, there are the
everyday interactions. The routines, tantrums, blank
stares, inappropiate behaviors are factors we have
grown to accept as part of the person we love.
We know, without understanding, the confinements
of our loved ones. We care for them, feed them,
bathe them, and give tolerance for their "unusual"
actions without expecting a great deal of loving
response.

The other half of the duality is the frustration we
feel at wondering what lies behind those stares, what
causes the tantrums, what abilities are locked up in the
beast that keeps them away from us. It's easy, and
very tempting, to romanticize the extent of their
knowledge and intelligence. It is just as human to
often underestimate the extent of their abilities. The
sad truth is that we may never know.

We all want so much to have them be normal,
to share in their dreams, to watch them reach career
goals, for them to have bonding male-female relations,
to one day play with their children. But, because we

realize that most of these dreams will not become realities, we accept the mystery and love the child.

It is so easy to dismiss what we do not understand. To stop trying to bring out the best in them, to not extend every day to reach a little further into the puzzle, is an easy answer that we, and they, cannot afford. The expense of wondering if we gave our best effort is far too costly.

However, there are hidden blessings. My father, I, and all the others that love Alex will never worry about him being on drugs, running with the wrong crowd, coming back home with two kids after a marriage breaks up, intentionally breaking laws or very importantly, not giving his best.

In many ways, the loved ones with autism in our lives have enriched us and made us stronger and more complete.

The challenge of autism, or maybe at times because of it, has made us love them all the more. Our hearts extend to embrace them as we understand that their handicap is, in fact, ours. We are prisoners in the mirror of autism; just as they can't reach us, we can't reach them in all the ways we'd like.

We long to find an easy answer to bring them out of their prisons. Simply put, it probably isn't there. There is not an instant cure, a magic panacea. The only answer is to give them our best and take great comfort from those small, but wonderful, victories that tell us that there is still hope and reason to keep trying.

If we ever take the easier path of just accepting their limits and not continuing to seek answers, then we will have thrown away the one key that may unlock the prison; we then would become the lonely ones ...forever.

Jennifer Gilpin
Maryland

"Alex"

After publication of the first book, many people have asked me to give more information on Alex. They seemed particularly interested in his progress the past year and his reaction to the book.

The latter first,... he doesn't give a flip! Simply put, Alex doesn't relate personally to the book other than understanding that it is partially about him. As best I can tell, the attendant hoopla doesn't affect him in an ego way. He did seem to like seeing his father on the television interview shows and was obviously pleased when one of the interviewers turned to the camera and thanked him for allowing his Dad to visit her.

He also went with me to one of the radio talk shows and enjoyed seeing the station operate and liked hearing me tell stories about him, as he sat in the waiting room adjacent to the booth.

But as far as being on the front page of the local paper, being recognized in school, etc. it was of little impact. I never worried about an inflated sense of importance. In fact, the truth is that I hoped that it would affect him that way somewhat. No, he just continued along, endearingly, as Alex, a sweet, gentle, non-threatening young man.

Now, to his progress. Alex is now going into the ninth grade, and is, for all intents and purposes, mainstreamed. For the first time, he is now going to classes without an aide, negotiating the locker-library classroom-cafeteria-restroom maze alone. I worry for his safety at times. He's so innocent and naive. Yet, other students seem to watch out for him and the chance of his being molested or bothered by bullies or malcontents seems to be relatively small.

This year he does his homework with little help. Alex gets out his books on time, follows the directions and, slowly, painstakenly and methodically completes his lessons.

Alex now does chores around the house and he does them well. He does dishes and takes out the trash. Alex rarely forgets and always follows through.

He has become even more of a pinball wizard. I often take him to the arcade where he amazes me with his dexterity and reflexes in maneuvering the ball around the various scoring mechanisms. To give the reader some idea of his skill, he recently played a machine where the level for a free game was pretty high, 42,000,000 points. Alex scored 232,400,000. My score was 14,000,000 and I thought I did pretty well.

As you may have seen in the book, he is developing a sense of humor, albeit very offbeat. Nevertheless, the important thing is that he is intentionally trying to be funny and delights when he makes people laugh. If he does something funny when he and I are alone, he will encourage me to tell others the humorous thing he said or did.

I've taken the time and space in this book to give you an in-depth view of Alex, circa 1994, because of those who've requested it, but more so, you, the reader who may be the parent, relative or teacher of a younger child with autism can see what the future may hold. The Alex of today would astound many professionals and honestly, family members, who had such gloomy predictions for his future when he was a small child.

There was talk of his not learning to read or write, that we should not expect very much interaction, that children with autism often had violent swings in personality and activity, and that we could expect regression at any time. I know that these do happen with some children with autism, but not to all and certainly without predictability.

Today, Alex is a young man who contributes to the happiness of those around him and takes joy from those that he loves. He sings in the school chorus, loves music, has reasonable social skills, is main-streamed in junior high school, and, most importantly, loves life.

Sometime, I'd like to find those "experts" who offered their sincere but misguided analysis, show them the Alex of 1994 and say, "never tell another parent that their child can't do, instead speak of what they can do; ...offer hope, not discouragement, ...resolve, not defeat, ...positives, not negatives. Never forecast limits, because you may cause them to become a reality."

To all of you who are dealing with the challenge of autism, I can't say it often enough or loudly enough.... never give up... never give up. These children and adults need you to be their biggest supporter and believer in them. I know it's tough at times, but your belief in his or her future is the seed for their improvement. Never, never stop believing that they can, and will be, better.

Never give up and, very importantly, ...keep smiling.